The MEMORY ROOM

A NEW WAY TO CREATE **CLARITY, CALM,** AND **CONNECTION** IN ASSISTED LIVING

MARK L. FOX

FOUNDER & INVENTOR, RESONA HEALTH

Mark L. Fox-- 1st ed.
Chief Editor, Shannon Buritz

ISBN: 978-1-954757-73-8
Remarkable Press

SENIOR CARE

HEALTH & MEDICINE

NEUROSCIENCE

Anyone who works in memory care has seen moments like these. There's the Tuesday when a resident who hasn't known their family for months suddenly says their name. Or the rare conversation that lasts a full twenty minutes. Sometimes, an eighty-three-year-old woman hears a favorite song and stands up to dance.

Those moments are not just luck. They happen when the brain returns to its best state of coordination. New research shows that these moments can happen more often, more reliably, and more intentionally than we once thought possible for dementia.

In *The Memory Room*, Resona Health founder Mark L. Fox draws on MIT's landmark 40 Hz Alzheimer's research, a completed Phase 1 clinical study, and the universal principles of energy exchange to make a carefully argued case: the cognitive variability that caregivers and families already observe in residents reflects real, measurable fluctuations in neural function and those fluctuations can be supported through a non-invasive, non-pharmacological approach that fits into any care facility's existing routine.

In a completed Phase 1 study, every participant showed measurable improvement in cognitive function. There were no regressions and no adverse effects. The results were highly statistically significant, with a confidence level of $p < 0.000001$. This book explains what these numbers mean for the people you care for, for their families, and for the future of memory care.

"My wife has advanced dementia. Daily use of the BlueVibe reduced the intensity, frequency, and duration of her agitation by approximately 40%. For myself, as her caregiver, that is a very large blessing. I have more patience and sleep more deeply."

– Jeffry P., Phase 1 Study Participant

"I enrolled my mother in the study. She's 83. After three weeks, she said she didn't feel depressed anymore. Her cognitive ability improved so much that I questioned whether this was my mother. She is ordering groceries on her phone and dancing to music."

– Joy P., Phase 1 Study Participant

For the caregivers who show up every morning.
And for the families who stay a little longer than they planned.
You already know what this book is about.

Contents

PART THREE

What Changes When Residents Improve

The Ripple Effects of Cognitive Support

PART FOUR

The Memory Room

What This All Means for the Future of Care

Foreword

Most families who come to memory care facilities carry both love and grief. They love the person who remains, still present in some ways, still able on some days to recognize and connect as before. At the same time, they grieve for the person who is slowly fading, as dementia gradually takes hold. The staff and caregivers in these places know these feelings well. They experience them daily, in every hallway and every conversation.

Mark Fox's book challenges a sense of resignation that has grown in memory care. This feeling does not come from indifference, but from the real belief that cognitive decline cannot be changed, so care is mostly about managing what cannot be fixed. While this belief is understandable, it is not the whole story. The difference between knowing dementia is progressive and thinking nothing can be done about daily life is important. This gap is where the most meaningful progress in the coming years can happen.

The science Fox shares in this book is real and respected, carried out by leading experts at top institutions. The MIT research on forty-hertz gamma stimulation is not fringe; it appears in top journals like *Nature* and *Cell* and has even surprised its own researchers. The BlueVibe Phase 1 study is a true clinical trial, not a marketing effort, and it produced real results. Fox's honest discussion of both the findings and the limits of this work shows why it deserves careful attention from everyone involved in caring for people with cognitive challenges.

For years, I have seen good interventions fail to reach those who needed them. The problem was not that these ideas did not work, but that the systems meant to review and use them moved too slowly and demanded too much proof before taking action. As a result, people missed out on help that was already possible. I hope this does not happen with the work described in this book. Please read it closely, judge it fairly, and then consider what the evidence asks you to do.

– Dr. Pedram Shojai
The Urban Monk

Introduction

I did not set out to write a book about memory care. I set out to build a better device, a device that could deliver forty-hertz electromagnetic stimulation to the brain in a form that was wearable, comfortable, and practical enough for daily use outside a laboratory. I had spent a career in aerospace engineering, working on systems where precision was not a preference but a requirement. The difference between a correctly specified signal and an incorrectly specified one could mean the difference between a successful mission and a catastrophic failure. When I began working in the field of frequency-based wellness technology, I brought that engineering discipline with me, and I applied it to a scientific question that I found genuinely fascinating: could the brain's own electrical rhythms be influenced from the outside, and if so, what would happen?

As you'll see in the following pages, the answer was more important than I expected. The science of forty-hertz gamma entrainment, which MIT researchers have studied carefully over the past decade, has big implications not just for device design, but for how we think about cognitive decline. The brain isn't just something that wears out. It's a dynamic electrical system that changes its coordination from day to day and hour to hour, affecting the person's experience. These changes can be influenced in meaningful ways by targeted stimulation at the right frequency, in the right way, and in the right place.

I wrote this book for people who run memory care facilities, manage their staff, and talk with the families who trust them with loved ones. The science I have worked with for years still hasn't become part of everyday care. This isn't because the science is weak, but because it takes a long time for research to reach daily practice. The people who need this knowledge most are often too busy running their facilities to dig into neuroscience journals. My goal with this book is to close that gap by sharing what is known, presenting it honestly, and making the case that it deserves real attention.

Here's how to use this book: It's meant to be read from start to finish, with each chapter building on the last. The first three chapters lay out the science: what cognitive variability is, what gamma oscillations mean for it, and what MIT research says about influencing it. The middle chapters cover the technology, show the clinical evidence, and answer practical questions about how to use it and what it costs. The final chapters focus on the ethical and human reasons for taking action. If you're short on time and want the main points, Chapters Five through Eight and the Appendices will give you the essentials. Still, I hope you'll read the whole book, since the argument is strongest when you see it all together.

I want to be clear, from the first pages of this book, about what I am not claiming. I am not claiming that BlueVibe cures Alzheimer's disease. I am not claiming that any device or technology can reverse the structural damage that dementia causes in the brain. The losses that cognitive decline produces are real, and they are not undone by the work described in this book. What I am claiming is more modest, and I believe it is more important for being modest: that the people living with those losses have more cognitive accessibility available to them than the current approach to care systematically supports, and that tools now exist to change that safely, practically, and at a cost that puts them within reach of any facility that takes the evidence seriously. That is the argument. I believe it. And I invite you to evaluate it for yourself.

– Mark L. Fox
Founder & Inventor, Resona Health,
Cocoa Beach, Florida, 2026

PART ONE

What We Already Know

Reframing the Problem Before Introducing the Solution

CHAPTER ONE

The Good Days

Why Families Call on Tuesdays

Memory care staff can often tell a certain kind of phone call not by the words, but by the tone. Caregivers who have worked in the facility for years notice these calls usually come on quieter days. The family member isn't calling to complain, report a fall, or ask about medication. Instead, they call because something good happened, and they aren't sure how to process it. Maybe their mother, who hasn't recognized them in months, looked up and said their name. Or their father, who rarely speaks in full sentences, told a story at dinner, a real story, with a beginning, middle, and end. Sometimes a grandmother holds a conversation for twenty minutes, asks questions, and laughs at the right times. After the visit, the family member drives home, replaying it in their mind, then calls the staff to ask whether what happened was real, whether they imagined it, and whether their loved one was, for a little while, more themselves.

The caregiver who answers that call knows, even if she can't always explain it, that these moments aren't as rare as families think. Good days do happen, and they happen fairly often in memory care, though not always for everyone or at predictable times. Staff learn to notice a certain brightness in a resident's face, a more alert posture, or a more thoughtful response to a greeting. Experienced caregivers pick up on these changes much like a teacher senses when a class is especially engaged, or a doctor can tell if a patient is truly well. This knowledge is real, but in most care settings, it hasn't been seen as something worth tracking.

This book starts with that observation: the good day, the unexpected visit, the family member who stayed much longer than planned, because it's the most honest way to begin asking questions the memory care field hasn't fully explored. What is really happening during these moments of greater clarity? Why does thinking, in people with real neurological damage, sometimes improve in ways that feel meaningful? And if these periods of lucidity and engagement are real, as every caregiver knows, what does that tell us about cognitive decline and what care can do?

Most people understand dementia as a gradual process of loss. Neurons die, networks break down, and over time, memory, language, and decision-making abilities fade. This view is accurate. The science supports it, and anyone who has cared for someone with advanced Alzheimer's knows these losses are real. This book does not dispute that. Instead, it asks a different, more focused question: for someone living with cognitive decline, what makes one day better than another? These days are not all the same, and the difference between them matters.

Think about how the field usually treats good days. People notice and appreciate them, and sometimes families record them in logs. Occasionally, these days are linked to something specific, like a visit, a favorite song, or a calming walk. More often, they are seen as unpredictable. There are many studies about decline in dementia, but far fewer about what helps people keep the abilities they still have. The important question of how to support the use of remaining cognitive skills has not received much attention, even though caregivers face it every day.

> *"I have noticed an improvement in my clarity of thinking and vocabulary words."*
>
> – Bonny F., Study Participant

A good day is not just a story to share. It shows that, even with serious brain changes, people can still have better or worse coordination in how their brain works. The fact that this ability changes from day to day is important. It means that a person with dementia does not always function at the same level. Instead, their brain can do more or less depending on the situation, and certain conditions can affect how well they do on any given day.

This way of looking at things does not suggest dramatic changes, and it is important to be clear about this. This does not mean that dementia can be reversed or that good days indicate someone is recovering. Instead, the point is that people at any stage of cognitive decline can have real differences in how well they function, and some of these differences are shaped by factors we can understand and possibly help. Good days are not just a matter of luck. They have neurological, environmental, and physical causes, and understanding those causes is both scientifically tractable and practically important.

This book will show that the ups and downs in thinking seen in people with dementia are partly due to how well their brain can coordinate activity in the networks that remain. This coordination can be improved with certain targeted, non-invasive methods. So, the important question is not just how to slow dementia's progress, but also how to help people with dementia use their minds as well as possible right now, wherever they are. Memory care workers have faced this question every day, and it is an important one to explore.

> *"I noticed better clarity and less stress."*
>
> – Susan R., Study Participant

CHAPTER TWO

The Brain We Thought We Knew

Why the Standard Story About Dementia Leaves So Much Unexplained

Many of us have a basic idea of what dementia does to the brain, even if no one has ever explained it to us. Neurons die, and the connections between them weaken and disappear. The parts of the brain responsible for memory, for example, the hippocampus and the frontal cortex, shrink over time. These changes can be seen on scans and measured with cognitive tests. This general understanding is mostly accurate and helps explain why recent memories fade before older ones, why finding words becomes harder, and why complex planning gets more difficult, even as some older skills and emotions remain. Scientists have recorded these brain changes well.

Even though the main model of dementia explains a lot, it struggles with something that doctors and caregivers see all the time: how much things can change from moment to moment.

If dementia were only about steady brain loss, you'd expect a smooth decline. But sometimes, a woman who can't remember her daughter's name at breakfast remembers it perfectly by dinner. A man who is quiet and withdrawn in the morning might be talkative and engaged later in the day. These changes happen too often to ignore. They show us that the usual model doesn't tell the whole story.

Part of the answer comes from a distinction that neuroscience has been exploring for years: the difference between the brain's structure and its function. Imagine a piano with some broken keys. That's a structural problem, a physical limit on what the piano can play. Now picture a concert pianist with severe arthritis trying to play a perfect piano. That's a functional problem: the piano is fine, but the performance changes depending on how the pianist feels. These are two different issues, and each needs a different kind of help. People with Alzheimer's disease face both permanent structural damage, like broken keys, and day-to-day changes in function, like the pianist's hands. The structural damage can't be fixed, but the functional changes can vary. This book focuses on those daily changes in how well the brain's remaining parts work together.

To see why this difference matters, it helps to understand how brainwaves work. You can think of the brain like a radio that tunes to different stations for different tasks. Deep sleep is like the lowest station, with slow, rolling delta waves that help you rest without dreams. Next are theta waves, which help with memory and light sleep. Alpha waves are like a relaxed FM station, the state you're in when you're calm but awake, such as when reading or walking. Beta waves are higher up, like a busy talk-radio station, and are linked to active cognition and reasoning. At the very top is gamma, the fastest brainwave, which the brain uses for its most complex and connected thinking.

Think about the last time you had a word on the tip of your tongue. You could almost sense it, the shape, maybe even the first letter, but the word just wouldn't come. Then, a few minutes later, it finally appeared. That whole process, from searching to finally finding the word, is an example of gamma at work. Gamma is the brain frequency that links and integrates information, pulling together pieces from different parts of the brain to form a complete thought. Things like forming and recalling memories, staying focused, thinking quickly, and recognizing a face, along with the feelings it brings, all rely on gamma coordination. Studies have shown that people with Alzheimer's disease and similar conditions often have disrupted or reduced gamma activity. This disturbance is consistent with cognitive symptoms: when gamma levels decline, coordination declines, and with less coordination, thinking becomes less clear.

Most people have had days when their thoughts just wouldn't come together. Maybe you walked into a room and forgot why, or read the same paragraph several times without understanding it, or couldn't remember a word you use all the time. These days often follow poor sleep, high stress, or not feeling well. On those days, your brain isn't damaged; the structure is the same as before. What's different is how well your brain's electrical signals are working. The gamma signal is weaker, the network isn't working smoothly, and thinking feels like trying to tune a radio with a weak signal. For people with Alzheimer's disease, this isn't just an occasional problem; it's their everyday experience. Still, the fact that some days are better than others, as many caregivers know, shows that electrical coordination can change and respond to different conditions. The structure of the brain doesn't change from one day to the next, but the signal quality does. Unlike structural damage, signal quality can be influenced.

Even with the structural damage caused by Alzheimer's disease, the brain still has a level of function that can change and respond to different conditions. This part of brain function can still be supported. The aim of care, then, is not to fix what is already lost, but to help people make the most of the abilities they still have. That is a goal worth working toward. As the next chapter shows, science is making this goal more achievable.

CHAPTER THREE

The MIT Discovery

What Happened When Scientists Flickered a Light at 40 Times per Second

In 2016, neuroscientist Li-Huei Tsai published a paper in *Nature* that, for a short time, attracted more public attention than most neuroscience research. The attention made sense. The study described what happened when MIT researchers exposed mice with Alzheimer's-like symptoms to light flickering exactly forty times per second. The results were something the field had tried and mostly failed to achieve with drugs: a big drop in amyloid-beta, the protein that forms Alzheimer's plaques. In the visual cortex of mice exposed to forty-hertz flickering light, amyloid-beta levels fell by about half compared to controls. Tau protein, another key sign of Alzheimer's, also dropped by a similar amount. The mice did better on cognitive tests, too. None of this involved drugs, surgery, or anything invasive. All it took was a light, flickering at a specific frequency, for an hour a day.

To see why this result was so important, it helps to know what amyloid-beta and tau are, and why decades of drug research have done little to control them. Imagine the brain's neural network as a complex plumbing system, with billions of pipes connecting everything. Amyloid-beta is like mineral buildup between the pipes, slowly narrowing them and blocking flow. If left alone, these deposits harden into the plaques that Alois Alzheimer first saw under a microscope over a century ago. Tau tangles are different: instead of building up between neurons, tau proteins go wrong inside them, causing the cell's internal support to collapse, much like a building's beams giving way. Both problems are real and harmful, and both have resisted drug treatments. Many drugs meant to clear amyloid-beta have failed to help thinking or have caused bad side effects. The plaques and tangles seemed out of reach for any safe treatment in living people.

The idea behind Tsai's experiment was simple, even if the science was not. Earlier research showed that gamma oscillations, forty-hertz electrical rhythms linked to memory, attention, and thinking, are disrupted in Alzheimer's disease. Tsai and her team at the Picower Institute for Learning and Memory studied this problem and asked a new question: if the brain's gamma rhythm is fading, what happens if you give it something to match? What if you used an outside signal, like light flickering forty times a second, and let the brain's rhythms sync up with it, just as someone might match their walking pace to a steady companion? The answer was yes, the brain does synchronize. And the effects of this were even bigger than the team expected.

The first and most striking effect was the activation of microglia, which are the brain's cleaning crew. Microglia are special immune cells that constantly patrol the brain, looking for debris and damage to clear away before it becomes a bigger problem. In a healthy brain, they are active and effective, like a cleaning team working all night. In a brain with Alzheimer's, they can become disorganized, sometimes overwhelmed or too slow to keep up. The MIT study found that forty-hertz stimulation got the cleaning crew moving again. It made microglia move toward amyloid plaques and improved their ability to clear away the buildup. The flickering light didn't bring a new drug into the brain. Instead, it signaled the janitors already there, and they got to work.

The second process involves the glymphatic system, which acts like the brain's dishwasher. Just as a dishwasher works best at night when nothing else is using water, the glymphatic system, a network that clears waste like amyloid-beta from the brain, mainly works during sleep. This is why poor sleep is now seen as a major risk for Alzheimer's: every bad night means the dishwasher didn't run, and waste builds up. The MIT study found that forty-hertz stimulation improved glymphatic flow. The flickering light seemed to help the brain's cleaning system work during the day, making up for the overnight cleaning that many older adults and memory care residents often miss. Since sleep problems are common in this group, this finding is important.

The third process involves maintaining synaptic connections. Think of synapses as the wiring in a house. Every memory, skill, or link between ideas and names exists as a real connection between two neurons. These are physical structures. When they break down, the memories and skills they held are lost too. You can have all your appliances, but if the wiring fails, nothing works. The number of healthy synaptic connections in key brain areas predicts thinking ability better than the number of amyloid plaques, because the wiring is what keeps everything running. The MIT study found that mice given forty-hertz stimulation kept far healthier synaptic connections than those without it. A therapy that slows synaptic loss is, quite literally, a therapy that keeps more of the lights on.

In a 2019 paper in *Cell*, the team added forty-hertz sound stimulation, a tone pulsed forty times per second, to their protocol. The results showed that this sound not only affected the auditory cortex but also the hippocampus. Combining visual and auditory stimulation at 40 Hz had effects across several brain regions simultaneously. They observed lower levels of amyloid-beta in the hippocampus and prefrontal cortex, reduced inflammation, and increased synaptic proteins. A 2021 human study in Alzheimer's and Dementia used both visual and sound stimulation in people with mild Alzheimer's. Over six months, these patients had much less brain shrinkage in memory areas than those who did not get the treatment. Multiple research groups have found similar results.

Forty-hertz stimulation is not just a theory or a wellness fad. It is a real therapeutic idea, supported by peer-reviewed studies in top journals such as *Nature* and *Cell,* as well as by growing evidence from human research. This approach is new in medicine, not by adding chemicals to the brain, but by bringing back the electrical rhythms the brain needs to stay healthy.

All the biological processes described here, the microglia cleaning, the glymphatic system's dishwasher, and the house's wiring are ways the brain protects itself. They show how the brain can be protected from further damage and, in some cases, even regain lost function. This is not the same as curing Alzheimer's, and it would be wrong to claim that. But it is the difference between a brain losing function with no help, and a brain losing function more slowly because it is getting support. For someone in memory care, for families, and for caregivers, that difference matters a lot. It is, in fact, the main point.

PART TWO

A New Kind of Support

From Understanding the Problem to Exploring the Tools

CHAPTER FOUR

What it Feels Like from the Inside

Listening More Carefully to What Residents Are Telling Us

Cognitive research relies on assessments that, by their nature, are somewhat limited. They measure what can be measured, such as how many words someone remembers after a delay, how quickly they match symbols, or how accurately they recall a date or a public figure's name. In the BlueVibe Phase 1 study, researchers used the PROMIS cognitive function tool, developed by the National Institutes of Health and widely recognized for its reliability. This tool asks people to rate their own memory, attention, processing speed, verbal fluency, and executive function. The results were impressive: every matched participant improved, no one got worse, and the statistics were highly significant, with a p-value less than 0.000001. Still, these numbers tell only part of the story. The rest comes from the words participants used to describe their experiences beyond the structured questions.

Think about what it means for someone to say, after six weeks of using a device for an hour each day, that they now have "clarity of thoughts." Their mind feels organized, ideas come easily, and thinking feels smooth instead of stuck. For someone who has struggled with cognitive problems, even a little clarity is a big deal. It gives them back a feeling of control. When a participant says they have clarity of thoughts, they are describing a real change in how they feel about themselves.

> *"I feel like the short-term memory was lengthened, so instead of forgetting things in about 5 or 10 minutes, it is more like hours, and even the next day. Also, my mood improved."*
>
> – Michael H., Study Participant

The participant who said their anxiety was "greatly reduced" was making a different but related point. Anxiety takes a toll on the mind. It uses up attention, disrupts memory, and makes it harder to recall information, sometimes making someone seem more impaired than they really are. When anxiety goes down not because of sedation, but in a way that leaves the person feeling more alert, the benefits for thinking and memory can be significant.

> *"It has helped me stay out of the dark places in my mind."*
>
> – Amber D., Study Participant

One story from the Phase 1 study stands out. A participant signed up their 83-year-old mother. After three weeks, the participant reported that their mother said she no longer felt depressed, a feeling neither of them had noticed until it was gone. It had just been part of her daily life: feeling flat, withdrawn, and uninterested in things. Once the depression lifted, they could see the difference. The participant said their mother's thinking and conversations improved so much that it was almost like she was a different person. She started ordering groceries online for the first time and even began dancing to music.

> *"I just want to repeat that the clarity and the depth of my thinking have improved, and my memory has improved somewhat. I had a severe concussion two years ago when I took a fall skiing at 30 miles an hour."*
>
> – Bonny F., Study Participant

One of the most interesting findings in the study is easy to miss: some participants did better on the cognitive tests but didn't feel any different themselves. When someone's scores go up, but they don't notice a change, it shows the improvement isn't just because they think they're getting better. These cases support the idea that the results are real and not just wishful thinking.

Taken together, these stories show that the effects of cognitive support are not the same for everyone. For some, it means clearer thinking. For others, it starts with feeling better emotionally. Sometimes, it shows up in new behaviors, like ordering groceries, dancing, or having conversations that surprise family members. These differences are a natural part of a complex and personal process: a brain, given the right support, finding its way back to working at its best.

CHAPTER FIVE

The Universal Exchange

Nothing Happens Without an Energy Exchange

Let's start with something familiar. Picture yourself at a campfire on a summer night. Someone hands you a stick with a marshmallow, and you hold it near the flames. The marshmallow softens, browns, and if you're not careful, it can burn at the edges. You press it between two graham crackers with a piece of chocolate, making a s'more, a simple, slightly silly treat that needs a campfire, a stick, some patience, and a clear night. But in that moment, you're also part of one of the universe's most basic processes: an energy exchange. The fire's heat travels through the air into the marshmallow. Its molecules absorb the energy, move faster, and begin to change. What was once a cold, white cylinder of sugar and gelatin becomes warmer, more complex, and more interesting. The only real change is that energy moved from one place to another. None of this would have happened without that exchange.

This isn't just a metaphor. It's a basic rule of how the physical world works, and once you notice it, you'll see that every event, big or small, is a kind of energy exchange. For example, if you step off a curb and miss, you feel a jolt as your body absorbs the energy from the fall. The bruise that appears later is your body's way of dealing with that energy hitting tissues that weren't ready for it. Or think about starting a car: you turn the key, a small electric pulse creates a spark, that spark ignites fuel, and the resulting gases push a piston, turning the crankshaft and moving the wheels. Every step in this process is an energy exchange, electrical, chemical, and mechanical, and none of it happens without energy moving from one form to another. If you spend a summer afternoon outside without sunscreen, you might end up with a sunburn. That's because your skin absorbed more light energy from the sun than it could handle. Sunburn isn't mysterious; it's simply what happens when living tissue takes in too much electromagnetic energy.

These examples all show something important that's easy to forget when thinking about therapy, medicine, or treating cognitive decline: the human body follows the same rules of energy exchange as everything else. Just like a marshmallow, a car, or your skin in the sun, our bodies are biological systems in a physical world that need energy to function. The body uses energy to function, reacts to energy from its surroundings, and suffers when it doesn't get the right kind or amount of energy. This is a basic fact of physiology. Once you see that the body runs on and responds to energy, it makes sense that applying energy to the body could have a therapeutic effect. It's simply a logical extension of a well-known principle.

So the real question isn't whether energy affects the body; it clearly does, all the time. The real question is which types of energy, delivered in what ways, and at what levels, are helpful rather than harmful. Researchers in energy therapy have found five main ways to deliver therapeutic energy to the body. Most people have experienced these in some form, even if they haven't thought about them as part of the same idea.

The first pathway is electrical current. Using direct electrical stimulation in medicine isn't new. The most common example is the TENS unit, which stands for transcutaneous electrical nerve stimulation. Millions of people use TENS units for pain relief, and physical therapists often recommend them. When you use a TENS unit, it sends an electrical current through your skin to target nerve pathways, either blocking pain signals or helping muscles work. This is energy therapy in its most straightforward form: electricity from a device enters the body and causes a clear biological response. It works because our bodies use electricity to communicate, so adding extra electrical signals can change how those systems work.

The second pathway is pulsed electromagnetic fields, or PEMF. This is the main method used by Resona Health for most of its devices, including BlueVibe. PEMF sends electromagnetic energy into the body without needing direct contact with the skin. The PEMF does not require direct skin contact, but the blue light does. So, for the BlueVibe to be most effective, it needs skin contact. There are no wires, sticky pads, or a need to plug into a wall. The energy travels from the device to the tissue, so you can wear it at the base of the neck or your wrist near vital meridian locations.

It works wherever you go. The therapy can continue during everyday activities, such as eating breakfast, taking a walk, or watching TV in a care facility, rather than requiring you to sit still and be hooked up to equipment. For older adults with limited mobility or who may not tolerate clinical procedures well, this portability makes regular daily use possible, and regular use is what leads to real therapeutic benefits.

The third pathway is light. Most people know light's harmful side, sunburn. But light can also be used for therapy. Red and near-infrared light therapy has extensive research supporting its ability to boost cellular energy, reduce inflammation, and aid tissue repair. Blue light at certain frequencies has been studied for its effects on sleep cycles and the brain. BlueVibe uses pulsed blue light as its second method, chosen for its ability to help with gamma entrainment. This means the light flickers at forty hertz, which MIT research found can help the brain's rhythms match those linked to memory and thinking. While sunburn is caused by excess light energy, the blue light from BlueVibe is delivered at a specific frequency and intensity, designed for a biological purpose and kept well below levels that could harm tissue.

The fourth pathway is vibration. The body reacts to mechanical vibration, which has been studied for its effects on bone strength, muscle function, and blood flow. Focused ultrasound, which uses high-frequency vibration aimed at specific tissues, is a well-known medical tool for imaging and therapy. In all these cases, mechanical energy at the right frequency and strength causes biological responses that can be measured and used for therapy.

The fifth pathway is sound. Sound, especially at certain frequencies, has been used in many therapies, from music therapy for dementia to specific sound frequencies in MIT's GENUS research. In 2019, MIT used forty-hertz tones pulsing forty times a second to help the brain's gamma rhythms in the hippocampus. Sound is simply mechanical pressure moving through air and tissue. Like the other energy forms, it can cause biological changes when the right frequency reaches the right tissue in the right amount.

All five pathways share the same basic idea: energy moves, and when it reaches living tissue, the tissue reacts. This is the same principle behind making a s'more, feeling a bruise after a fall, driving a car, or getting sunburned. In energy therapy, the key scientific question is about precision, figuring out exactly which type of energy, delivered in what way, causes which response in which tissue.

When looking at how energy therapy works at the cellular level, scientists agree on two main ways it helps. The first is about the electrical charge of each cell. Every living cell has a measurable voltage across its membrane, and this voltage is important. It controls how nutrients enter the cell and how waste leaves. You can think of it like a car battery: a fully charged battery works well, but a low battery struggles and can't do its job. The same goes for cells. When a cell's voltage is within the healthy range, usually between 70 and 100 millivolts, it takes in nutrients and expels waste efficiently. If the voltage drops because of illness, aging, stress, or injury, the cell can't do these jobs as well. Nutrients stay outside, waste builds up inside, and the cell just isn't working at full power. Studies show that PEMF can raise the voltage across cell membranes, basically recharging the cell and helping it work better.

The second way energy therapy helps is through ATP, or adenosine triphosphate. If the cell's voltage is like its electrical charge, ATP is the fuel that powers everything the cell does. ATP stores and moves energy inside the cell and is needed for almost every process. When there's plenty of ATP, cells work well. When ATP is low, cells slow down, repair less, and the body can't keep up with its needs. This is especially important for the brain, which uses about twenty percent of the body's energy. Brain cells that don't have enough energy can't fire properly, keep their connections, or coordinate the fast activity needed for memory and thinking. Research from many groups has shown that PEMF can boost ATP production in cells by up to five hundred percent. This is a big, repeatable increase in the main fuel supply for the cells the device targets.

When you combine these two effects, you get a clear picture of how energy therapy works at the cellular level. It raises the voltage on the cell membrane, helping cells take in nutrients and remove waste more efficiently. It also boosts ATP, giving cells more fuel to do their jobs. These changes don't cure Alzheimer's or fix lost brain cells, but they do help the remaining cells work better by giving them more energy and resources. This is how energy therapy supports the body's natural ability to heal itself when it has what it needs.

CHAPTER SIX

The Body's Own Signals

How BlueVibe Puts These Principles to Work

When senior living administrators first hear the term "pulsed electromagnetic field therapy," they often respond with polite caution. The phrase itself can sound intimidating. "Electromagnetic" might bring to mind heavy machinery or radiation warnings. This chapter does not aim to dismiss those concerns, but instead to put them in perspective, building on the previous chapter's point that energy exchange is a normal part of how the world works. Every physical and biological event relies on it. PEMF is simply a precise, controlled, and non-invasive way to deliver a specific type of energy to the brain's electrical systems. To visualize this, imagine striking a tuning fork and holding it near a piano string tuned to the same note. The string starts to vibrate, not because it was touched, but because the energy in the air matched its natural frequency. This is called resonance, a basic idea in physics. PEMF works in a similar way: it sends pulsed electromagnetic energy at forty hertz, which corresponds to the brain's gamma frequency, and encourages the brain's systems to sync, just like the piano string responds to the tuning fork.

Pulsed electromagnetic field therapy has been used in clinical settings longer than many people think. In 1979, the United States Food and Drug Administration approved PEMF devices for the treatment of non-union bone fractures, based on solid clinical evidence from controlled trials. The way PEMF works is similar to wireless phone charging: a device creates an electromagnetic field, and nearby tissue, like a phone on a charging pad, absorbs the field and turns it into cellular activity. There are no wires, adhesive pads, or direct contact with a power source. The energy travels through space and is absorbed by the body at levels much lower than those of any household electronic device. The FDA's approval in 1979 marked the start of decades of heightened recognition that electromagnetic field stimulation is a real and effective therapy for living tissue.

It's important to highlight the engineering behind Resona Health's approach. The company's device platform was built using aerospace engineering principles, thanks to a founding team with experience in high-stakes environments where accuracy is critical. Their focus on exact signal delivery, consistency, and controlled performance sets their therapeutic device apart from general wellness gadgets that use electromagnetic fields. When frequency, intensity, and pulse timing are accurately set and delivered, the body receives reliable, measurable stimulation. If not, the results can vary widely.

BlueVibe provides stimulation at forty hertz using two

methods: pulsed electromagnetic energy and pulsed blue light, both set to the same frequency. This paired approach is based on MIT research showing that using two stimulation pathways at once, like playing the same note on two instruments, activates more of the brain's network than using just one. The device is worn at the base of the neck, close to the brainstem and the vagus nerve, which are important for regulating stress, emotions, and neurological signals. This area is also linked to cerebrospinal fluid flow, which helps clear waste from the brain, as explained in the previous chapter.

> *"How easy, inconspicuous, and comfortable it is to use."*
>
> – John M., Study Participant

> *"Easy to use and relaxing."*
>
> – Thomas B., Study Participant

PEMF is not the same as ionizing radiation or the types of electromagnetic exposure known to damage tissue. The electromagnetic spectrum covers a wide range, and each part acts differently. X-rays and gamma rays, for example, have enough energy to break chemical bonds, which is why their use is strictly controlled. In contrast, the fields used in therapeutic PEMF are at the very low end of the spectrum, much lower than visible light or even the radio waves emitted by a mobile phone, and at strengths much weaker than the body's own electrical activity. Saying PEMF is dangerous just because it uses electromagnetic fields is like saying a whisper is dangerous because sound can harm hearing. What matters are the frequency and intensity, and both are carefully chosen to help, not harm, the body's systems.

It's reasonable for a skeptical administrator to wonder: if this technology is effective and well-supported, why isn't it already standard in memory care? Even proven new therapies take time to become common in healthcare. The process from research to regular use through publication, replication, updating guidelines, training, and adoption can be slow. Facilities that start using tools like BlueVibe early are not being reckless. Instead, they are focusing on real evidence, safe technology, and an important clinical need that is often overlooked.

CHAPTER SEVEN

The Study

What 41 People and a Six-Week Trial Can (And Cannot) Tell Us

Sometimes people read clinical research by focusing only on the headline number and making quick judgments. For example, a one hundred percent improvement rate might seem impressive at first glance. But this approach misses important context. Numbers like these need to be understood in light of the study's design, the group of people involved, the statistical methods used, and an honest look at what the results do and do not prove. A headline that holds up under close examination is much more valuable than one that has not been questioned. The BlueVibe Phase 1 study is strong enough to deserve that closer look.

The study followed a within-subject, pre- and post-intervention design. Forty-one people took a baseline cognitive test and then took the same test again after about six weeks of using the device. The test used was the PROMIS Cognitive Function scale from the National Institutes of Health. Participants used the

BlueVibe device in their everyday lives for about an hour each day. There was no lab setting, no controlled environment, and no daily clinical supervision. This approach tested the device in real-world conditions, which is a real strength of the study's design.

The results all pointed in the same direction. Every one of the forty-one participants improved their overall cognitive function score from the first test to the follow-up. Not just most of them, all of them. No one got worse. To put this in perspective, imagine flipping a coin forty-one times and getting heads every time. The odds of that happening by chance are less than one in two trillion. The BlueVibe study saw the same kind of unlikely pattern: forty-one people, forty-one improvements, none in the opposite direction. The researchers used the paired Wilcoxon signed-rank test, which is the appropriate method for this kind of data, and found a p-value of < 0.000001. In simple terms, the chance that these results occurred by chance is less than 1 in a million. In clinical research, a result is considered statistically significant if the p-value is below 0.05, or one in twenty. This study's result is fifty thousand times more significant than that standard.

You might wonder how such strong statistical confidence is possible with only forty-one participants. Here's one way to think about it: if you want to know if it will rain tomorrow, a forecast of 60% chance of rain from a thousand weather stations is helpful but not certain. But if forty-one independent weather stations all predict a 100% chance of rain, that's much more convincing. Statistical power depends not just on the number of observations, but also on how consistent they are. When all forty-one results point in the same direction, it creates a pattern that is very unlikely to be due to chance.

It's important to be clear about what this study cannot prove. Because it used a pre/post design without a control group, it cannot rule out other possible explanations for the observed improvements. The Phase 1 study was meant to test real-world use and look for signals, not to be a final, definitive trial. What Phase 1 shows is a clear, consistent, and statistically significant pattern: all 41 weather stations agree on rain. Whether BlueVibe alone caused this effect or whether other factors played a role is something that Phase 2 controlled research will need to answer. Phase 1 provides a strong reason to move forward with the next step.

The study's findings about perception and measurement are especially important. Some participants showed clear improvement on tests, even though they did not feel any different themselves. This is one of the study's most convincing results. A true placebo effect depends on people believing they are getting better. If someone's scores improve but they don't feel it, the improvement can't be explained by their expectations. They didn't think they were improving, but they did anyway. That matters.

Among the forty-one participants who used the device for about an hour each day over six weeks, no one reported any negative side effects. This is a valuable finding, especially since many people in this group often take several medications, have other health conditions, and may be more physically vulnerable because of age. It means the device can be offered to residents without the need for extra monitoring, complicated dosing, or managing side effects like with medications.

> *"My wife has advanced dementia. One of her disturbing symptoms is aggressive behavior, like slamming doors and general agitation. Daily use of the BlueVibe seems to have reduced the intensity, frequency, and duration of these behaviors. I would estimate it to be approximately 40%. For myself, as her caregiver, that is a very large blessing. I have more patience and sleep more deeply."*
>
> – Jeffry P., Study Participant

To sum up, the BlueVibe Phase 1 study shows a clear, statistically remarkable pattern of consistent improvement, a perfect safety record over six weeks, and a device that people found easy and comfortable to use. This is not the final answer, but it is a very strong start. It deserves the careful, thorough follow-up this book recommends.

CHAPTER EIGHT

The Simplicity Principle

Why the Most Effective Interventions Are Often the Easiest to Sustain

Some ideas seem promising in conference presentations but do not work in real care facilities. The research might be strong, the clinical reasoning solid, and the pilot data encouraging. But when an intervention meets a busy Tuesday morning with staff shortages, family concerns, and several residents needing help at once, it often gets set aside. Staff do not stop using these interventions because they do not care or lack skill. They stop because the intervention was not designed for the real challenges of a typical day. Implementation science calls this problem implementation decay.

Noticing implementation decay is needed to create interventions that actually work. The main question is not just whether an intervention helps in perfect clinical settings. It is whether it works in real situations, with real staff, busy schedules, and many demands. The benefit should also last beyond the first few weeks and continue through months of daily use.

BlueVibe was made to solve this problem. There are no apps to install, no need for Wi-Fi, and no software to learn. The device has one button. Press it to start, place it on the person's neck, and that is it; it automatically shuts off after a 1-hour session. Each session lasts an hour, and then the device is ready for the next resident. The process is simple enough to explain in one sentence because it was designed to be that easy.

> *"Helping my sleep every night without taking melatonin."*
>
> – Flora W., Study Participant

> *"It's simple to use. I also believe it has helped me to dream and remember dreams."*
>
> – Carolyn H., Study Participant

BlueVibe uses a shared-device model instead of giving every resident their own unit. In a facility, ten devices are rotated among twenty to forty or more residents each day. At the current wholesale price, the total daily cost for the whole facility is about $1.60.

The device is a lightweight band worn around the neck, with a small module at the base of the neck. It was designed to be comfortable so using it feels easy, not like a chore. If a device is bulky, obvious, or uncomfortable, people will not want to use it. Many participants said they forgot they were wearing it after about ten seconds.

How staff respond is likely the most important part of making this work. BlueVibe does not require clinical training, certification, or supervised practice. Any staff member can put the device on a resident, press the button, and collect it an hour later after a short introduction. The device does not change the clinical workflow. Instead, it fits into daily routines without making staff change how they work.

The Simplicity Principle does not mean choosing convenience over clinical quality. In fact, it is a kind of clinical wisdom. An intervention that is used regularly with many residents gives more overall benefit than one that is theoretically better but too hard to use in practice.

PART THREE

What Changes When Residents Improve

The Ripple Effects of Cognitive Support

CHAPTER NINE

The Ripple Effect

When One Person in the Room Feels Calmer, Everyone Does

Memory care facilities are emotional ecosystems. The moods, behaviors, and states of individual residents do not stay within their own rooms or bodies. Instead, they move through shared spaces, affect others nearby, and shape the overall atmosphere in ways that experienced caregivers notice right away. When a resident is very agitated, such as shouting in the hallway, resisting care, or moving through the common room in distress, the impact on others is clear and immediate. The disruption spreads through the environment, and its effects can be felt even far from where it started.

The opposite is also true. In a unit where most residents are calm, engaged, and able to interact socially, the atmosphere feels different. Experienced administrators can sense this as soon as they walk in. Staff move with less tension and more presence, focusing on meaningful care instead of always preparing for a crisis. Families notice the difference too, even if they cannot always explain exactly what feels better.

There is a lot of research on caregiver burnout. The most stressful parts of memory care work are the behavioral and psychological symptoms of dementia, like agitation, aggression, wandering, and resistance to care. Staff who often deal with these challenges report more emotional exhaustion, more secondary traumatic stress, and are more likely to want to leave their jobs than those who spend more time building relationships with residents. When residents are less agitated, staff can focus on the work that brought them to this field in the first place: building relationships, having conversations, and making real connections with people facing tough challenges.

> *"For myself, as her caregiver, that is a very large blessing. I have more patience and sleep more deeply."*
>
> – Susan R., Study Participant

Family satisfaction is just as important when residents show better cognition, because families are central to memory care. Families of people with dementia are often some of the most anxious people in any healthcare setting. When they see real improvement during their visit and find their loved one more present, more talkative, and more able to join in conversation, they change too. They become advocates rather than critics, and ambassadors rather than monitors.

> *"I have been calmer and sleeping better."*
>
> – Linda C., Study Participant

> *"Improved sleep and mood."*
>
> – Nancy P., Study Participant

A resident who is more present, who can have a short conversation, respond to a greeting with recognition, and join morning activities with real interest, is someone with whom a meaningful relationship is possible. Caregivers who spend their shifts truly interacting with residents experience their work differently than those who spend their time just managing behaviors and doing tasks. When this kind of work is possible, the job becomes more sustainable, and the facility is more likely to keep its experienced staff.

The Phase 1 study shows that when residents' cognitive function and emotional regulation improve in a consistent way, these positive effects are more likely to happen. Calmer residents lead to calmer units. Calmer units are less stressful for staff. When staff are not worn out by constant crises, they can focus more on building relationships with residents. While none of these results are guaranteed, they are much more likely when residents are regularly supported to be at their best, instead of leaving it up to chance.

CHAPTER TEN

The Cost of Doing Nothing

A Frank Conversation About Resources, Risk, and What We Owe Our Residents

Budget discussions in senior living usually follow a set pattern. New expenses are compared to current budget items, judged by their immediate cost, and approved or rejected based on short-term financial sense. But this approach often misses something important: it clearly shows the cost of taking action, but not the cost of doing nothing. The ongoing cost of the problem an expense could solve is hidden in the baseline, such as the staff hours spent managing behaviors, the cost of medications and monitoring, and the time spent talking with concerned families.

Staff time is the biggest and most often underestimated cost in memory care. When a resident's cognitive symptoms are not well managed, they use staff time in unpredictable ways, often interrupting care for others. If a caregiver spends twenty minutes calming a resident, that is also twenty minutes when other residents miss their scheduled care.

Using medication to manage behavioral and psychological symptoms of dementia is the usual approach. Antipsychotic drugs are most often used for agitation and other symptoms, even though they have a black box warning for elderly patients with dementia and are linked to higher risks of stroke, heart problems, and death. The cost of managing these drugs, including monitoring, paperwork, doctor oversight, and talking with families, often exceeds the price of the medication itself. The shift toward non-drug approaches is not about ideology. It comes from a realistic look at the true costs of medication and what families and regulators now expect instead.

> *"Seemed to brighten my mood."*
>
> – Ron J., Study Participant

In this context, BlueVibe's costs are simple to understand. The system, which includes 10 devices, costs $1,749 at current wholesale prices, over 50% less than retail. Used daily for twenty to forty residents, the total daily cost is about $1.60 for the whole facility, not per resident. The devices are built to last for years and require no additional supplies or subscriptions, so the yearly cost is small enough to barely affect most facility budgets.

> *"Hope for improvement."*
>
> – Paula S., Study Participant

If a facility can show with clinical data that a non-drug cognitive support program leads to real improvements in residents' cognitive function, it stands out in a meaningful way. Families choosing care are more informed and demanding than they were ten years ago. When a family sees real results, their recommendation is more valuable than any marketing effort.

PART FOUR

The Memory Room

What This All Means for the Future of Care

CHAPTER ELEVEN

The Ethics of Possibility

When a Tool Exists That Might Help, What Does Inaction Mean?

Clinical inertia is a common issue in healthcare, where people keep using the same practices even when new evidence points to better options. It's a system problem, and recognizing it is the first step toward real improvements. When we look at non-drug treatments in geriatric care, a pattern stands out. Music therapy, for example, was once met with both support and skepticism, just as newer methods like PEMF are today. Now, music therapy is strongly supported by evidence and recommended in dementia care guidelines. Other treatments, such as reminiscence therapy, physical activity, and bright-light therapy, followed the same process: initial doubt, more evidence, gradual adoption, and finally acceptance as good practice.

Risk asymmetry helps explain what is happening here. BlueVibe has a low risk profile. In Phase 1, no adverse effects were reported, and the device is non-invasive, not a drug, and easy to stop using. If a resident tries it and does not benefit, they only spend an hour wearing a comfortable device. If they do benefit, they get something that current care cannot provide.

> *"I enjoyed using it and felt more relaxed."*
>
> – Karen L., Study Participant

> *"I felt more focused while using it."*
>
> – Barbara T., Study Participant

This intervention is comfortable, non-invasive, easy to stop, and has a strong safety record backed by good evidence. These features make it easier to talk about with families. When families are asked if they want their parent to join a program using a comfortable wearable device, supported by a clinical study showing full improvement and no side effects, they have a positive option to consider.

From an ethical point of view, we do not need complete certainty right now. Medicine almost never gives us total certainty, and waiting for it can lead to inaction. Instead, ethics require a balanced response that matches the strength of the evidence, the size of the need, and the risks involved.

The best way to respond to Phase 1 evidence is not to use the intervention without thought or to put it off forever. A pilot program gives a set time for structured use, with assessments before and after, staff training, family updates, and careful tracking of results. If a resident improves during a BlueVibe pilot, they are not just a data point. They are a person in a facility where someone decided to try a promising tool. The ethics behind that choice are simple: they are the ethics of care.

CHAPTER TWELVE

The Memory Room

What We Are Really Talking About When We Talk About Clarity

Think back for a moment to that Tuesday afternoon. The phone rings, and the family member is gently and honestly told that yes, what they saw was real. For a while that day, their loved one was more present than they had been in months. The caregiver who answers does not go into detail. She does not have the words to explain what happened or why, or how to make it happen again. She says what experienced caregivers know to say: good days happen, she is glad it was a good day, and she hopes the family will visit again soon. The family member hangs up feeling something hard to name, not quite hope, but something close. A kind of quiet gratitude.

The Memory Room in this book's title is not a real place. It is a state of mind that some people with cognitive decline can sometimes reach, where memory, attention, and language come together again, even if only for a short time. Things are not fully restored, but they are gathered enough. Gathered enough for a conversation to last twenty minutes. Gathered enough for a name to come when needed. Gathered enough for an eighty-three-year-old woman to hear a song she likes in another room, walk toward it, and dance. Every caregiver who has worked in memory care for more than a year has seen someone reach this state, and they always recognize it right away.

> *"Better concentration. Better sleep. More dreams."*
>
> – Christine S., Study Participant

What this book has tried to do, across the chapters that preceded this one, is to give that recognition a more complete vocabulary. We have explored the neuroscience of gamma oscillations and their role in cognitive function. We reviewed the MIT research showing that 40 Hz stimulation is a credible therapy, including its effects on amyloid-beta, microglial activity, glymphatic function, and synaptic health. We discussed how energy exchange shapes the physical world and the body, and explained the five ways therapeutic energy can be delivered, along with the two main cellular effects: increased membrane voltage and more ATP production. We also looked at a clinical study with 41 participants, in which all participants improved, none regressed, and no negative effects were reported after 6 weeks of daily use. We learned that the conditions which produce better days are not random, that they are susceptible to influence by non-invasive means, and that the technology to do this influencing now exists in a form that is practical enough, safe enough, and supported by evidence strong enough to warrant serious and structured attention from anyone responsible for the cognitive care of an aging population.

Think about what it means, both practically and personally, for a resident to spend more time in that state. It means conversations with a more real connection, not just going through the motions. It means taking part in the small routines of daily life, choosing a favorite chair, enjoying a familiar meal, or making a decision instead of just accepting what is given. These moments help keep a sense of self, even when memory and language are fading. It also means a family member visits on a Wednesday, finds their loved one present, stays longer than planned, and leaves feeling something other than sadness.

There is one last story from the Phase 1 study to share. A participant decided to stop using the device for a week as a personal experiment to see if it really made a difference. After a week without it, they wrote: "I stopped using my device for a week and realized how much it was actually helping." This person did not expect to benefit at first. They conducted their own test, observed the result, and reached a careful conclusion. The device was helping. Its absence was clear.

> *"It gave me more energy during the day."*
>
> – James K., Study Participant

Facilities that start using BlueVibe in the coming months and years will be doing what the best facilities always do: paying close attention to what their residents need, finding the right tools, and using them with care and thoughtfulness. They will not offer a cure or make promises that science cannot support. Instead, they will be doing something more valuable and realistic: creating the conditions that help people in their care visit the Memory Room more often, in a state of gathered attention and presence that every caregiver knows and every family member hopes for. The Tuesday phone call will still happen, but maybe more often. And over time, the caregiver who answers may have better words to explain what occurred. Not luck. Conditions. And conditions can be created.

Acknowledgments

This book owes everything to the forty-one people who took part in the BlueVibe Phase 1 study. They shared their time, honest feedback, and often their personal stories, some of which are quoted in these pages, to help us find out if this technology works. Their openness to trying a new device and carefully reporting what they experienced is the reason this book exists. I am deeply grateful to each of them.

I am also thankful for the memory care professionals who took this work seriously. The administrators asked tough questions, the directors of nursing pushed for solid answers, and the caregivers on the floor shared what really happens in a facility early in the morning. Their practical knowledge shaped BlueVibe's design and this book's writing. The Simplicity Principle in Chapter Eight is here because of what they taught us.

The scientific community whose work supports this book, especially the researchers at MIT's Picower Institute for Learning and Memory, deserves recognition for its important contributions. Their careful, repeatable findings on forty-hertz gamma entrainment provided this project with its scientific foundation. Li-Huei Tsai and her colleagues are mentioned in these pages because their work has made a real difference in understanding the biology of Alzheimer's disease.

To the team at Resona Health: your dedication to precise engineering, honest evidence, and the belief that technology can help people without losing rigor or accessibility made this work possible. And to my family, who have heard more about pulsed electromagnetic fields and gamma oscillations than they ever expected to, thank you for listening.

APPENDIX A

The Phase 1 Study

A Summary for Clinical Review

This appendix provides a condensed technical summary of the BlueVibe Phase 1 clinical study for medical directors, clinical consultants, and others who wish to review the evidence directly. It is written for a clinically literate reader and assumes familiarity with standard research terminology.

Background

BlueVibe is a wearable, non-invasive therapeutic device that delivers dual-modality stimulation at 40 Hz: pulsed electromagnetic field energy and pulsed blue light, both oscillating at the same frequency. The device is worn at the posterior neck (occipital/upper cervical region) for approximately one hour per session. The 40 Hz frequency target is informed by a growing body of research, primarily from MIT's Picower Institute for Learning and Memory, demonstrating that gamma-frequency entrainment reduces amyloid-beta accumulation, activates microglial clearance, enhances glymphatic function, and preserves synaptic connectivity in preclinical models and early human trials.

Study Design

Phase 1 used a within-subject, pre-/post-intervention design without a control group. This design is appropriate for an initial feasibility and signal-detection study. It cannot establish causation in the strict scientific sense, and results should be interpreted in that context. Participants completed a baseline cognitive assessment and a follow-up assessment approximately 6 weeks after real-world device use. There was no clinical supervision of individual sessions; participants used the device in normal daily life conditions.

Population

Forty-one matched participant pairs were included in the analysis. Incomplete responses were excluded. Name inconsistencies and duplicate entries were resolved prior to analysis. Only valid pre/post matched pairs were included in the statistical analysis. The study population included adults using the device for cognitive support in real-world settings.

Assessment Instrument

The PROMIS Cognitive Function scale (Patient-Reported Outcomes Measurement Information System) was used. PROMIS instruments are developed and validated by the National Institutes of Health and are widely used in published clinical research. The cognitive function scale assesses memory, attention and concentration, mental clarity, processing speed, verbal fluency, and executive function. Responses are aggregated into a composite score, allowing pre/post comparison.

Results

41 of 41 matched participants (100%) showed improvement in composite cognitive function score from baseline to follow-up. 0 participants showed regression. 0 adverse effects were reported across the study period. The 100% improvement rate, with zero regressions across all matched participants, represents a uniformly positive directional signal.

Statistical Analysis

A paired Wilcoxon signed-rank test was applied. This is a non-parametric method appropriate for paired ordinal/non-normally distributed data. Result: $p < 0.000001$. Statistical confidence: >99.9999%. The probability that the observed uniform improvement pattern occurred by chance is less than 1 in 1,000,000. The extraordinary statistical confidence is a function of effect consistency (100% directional uniformity) rather than sample size alone.

Safety and Tolerability

No adverse effects were reported by any participant during the six-week study period. Device tolerability was high: participants reported the device as comfortable, easy to operate, and non-intrusive during normal daily activities. The device requires no skin adhesion, no electrical contact, no user calibration, and no clinical oversight for daily use.

Limitations

The absence of a randomized control group means that causal attribution to the device cannot be established with certainty from Phase 1 data alone. Alternative explanations, such as natural variation, expectation effects, and environmental changes during the study period, cannot be fully excluded. Phase 2 investigation with an appropriate controlled design is warranted and planned. The finding that several participants showed measurable improvement without subjective perception of benefit reduces (though does not eliminate) the likelihood that expectation effects account for the observed signal.

Conclusion

The BlueVibe Phase 1 study demonstrates a consistent, statistically extraordinary signal of cognitive improvement across all study participants, with a perfect safety record and high device tolerability. These findings constitute an appropriate justification for Phase 2 investigation and for structured facility use under monitored conditions.

APPENDIX B

Frequently Asked Questions from Facility Directors

The following questions have been compiled from conversations with memory care administrators, directors of nursing, and clinical consultants evaluating BlueVibe for facility use. They represent the most common practical concerns raised by people considering the pilot program.

Can BlueVibe be used if the participant has a pacemaker ?

As with any PEMF device, you should not use this device if you have a pacemaker, implanted defibrillator, neurostimulator, insulin pump, cochlear implant, or any other implanted electronic medical device. PEMF fields may interfere with the operation of implanted electrical devices. If used with any of the above, do so only under direct physician observation.

How do we explain BlueVibe to families?

Most families respond well to a straightforward explanation: BlueVibe is a wearable device that delivers gentle electromagnetic and light stimulation at a specific frequency associated with brain health. It is non-invasive, has no side effects, and takes about an hour to use. A completed clinical study showed that 100% of participants improved their cognitive function scores, with no adverse effects reported. Families who understand that this is a non-drug, evidence-based addition to their person's care, not a replacement for existing treatment, typically receive it positively.

Does the device require individual consent from residents?

The same consent standards that apply to other non-clinical wellness interventions in your facility apply to BlueVibe. For residents who can provide informed consent, a brief explanation and agreement are appropriate. For residents who cannot, the decision should be made in consultation with the resident's legal representative or healthcare proxy, applying the facility's standard best-interest or substituted judgment framework. The device's risk profile: zero adverse effects, easy discontinuation, and non-invasive nature make the consent conversation considerably simpler than for pharmacological interventions.

How is the device cleaned between residents?

The device should be wiped down between uses with standard disinfectant wipes appropriate for electronic devices. The neck band is designed for easy cleaning. Resona Health can provide guidance on specific cleaning protocols. The shared-device model is similar to other shared assistive technology in care environments and does not require more elaborate infection control procedures than are already standard in your facility.

What training do staff need?

Minimal. The device has one button. Staff need to understand how to place the device correctly on the resident's neck (the module sits at the base of the neck against the skin), how to start a session, and how to clean the device between uses. A brief orientation, typically 15 to 20 minutes, is sufficient for most staff members to use the device confidently. No clinical training, certification, or ongoing supervision protocol is required.

What if a resident refuses to wear the device?

Participation should always be voluntary. If a resident refuses or becomes agitated when the device is applied, remove it and document the response. Some residents may be more receptive on different days or at different times of day. Staff discretion in reading resident readiness is appropriate. The device's tolerability data from Phase 1 study participants showed that participants forgot they were wearing it after about 10 seconds, suggesting that initial resistance often resolves once the resident has worn it.

How many sessions per week do residents need?

The Phase 1 study used approximately one hour of daily use. For facility implementation, a protocol of five to seven sessions per week is recommended for residents who tolerate the device well. Facilities with scheduling constraints may find that three to four sessions per week still produce meaningful benefit, though the evidence base for specific dosing frequencies is still being developed. Consistent use over weeks is more important than any specific per-week frequency.

How does the pilot program work?

The pilot program runs for thirty to forty-five days. Before the pilot begins, participating residents complete a baseline PROMIS Cognitive Function assessment. The same assessment is administered at the end of the pilot period. Resona Health provides the assessment instrument and support for administering it. At the conclusion of the pilot, you receive an outcome summary report that shows pre- and post-scores for your resident population, providing facility-specific data to inform your decision on ongoing wholesale adoption.

What does the research base look like beyond the Phase 1 study?

The scientific foundation for 40 Hz stimulation as a therapeutic approach extends well beyond the BlueVibe study. The MIT Picower Institute research program on gamma entrainment includes multiple peer-reviewed publications in *Nature*, *Cell*, and other leading journals, demonstrating amyloid-beta reduction, microglial activation, glymphatic enhancement, and synaptic preservation in preclinical models, and early human trials showing reduced brain atrophy and preserved cognitive function. Appendix C of this book provides a reference guide to the key published research. PEMF has specifically been studied in more than 40 published studies across a range of applications. The FDA cleared PEMF devices for bone healing in 1979, and the modality has an established safety record over more than four decades of clinical use.

Can BlueVibe be used alongside existing medications and treatments?

Yes. BlueVibe does not interact with medications. It does not require the discontinuation of any existing treatment. It is not contraindicated with any common medication class used in memory care. As with any new addition to a resident's care routine, it is appropriate to document its introduction in the care record and to note any observed changes.

What happens after the pilot, and how does wholesale pricing work?

Facilities that complete the pilot program are eligible for wholesale pricing of more than 50% off retail. Resona Health provides ongoing facility support, including replacement devices, cleaning protocols, updated assessment resources, and access to new research as it is published. The wholesale relationship is designed as a long-term partnership rather than a transactional sale; the goal is to support facilities in integrating BlueVibe into their standard of care over time.

APPENDIX C

The Science of 40 Hz Gamma Stimulation

A Reference Note

This appendix provides a reference-level overview of the scientific literature on 40 Hz gamma stimulation and its relevance to Alzheimer's disease and cognitive decline. It is intended for readers who wish to explore the research in more depth than the main text provides, and for medical directors and clinical consultants who want to evaluate the scientific foundation independently.

Gamma Oscillations and Alzheimer's Disease

Gamma oscillations (30-100 Hz, with 40 Hz as the primary focus of research) are high-frequency neural oscillations associated with cognitive binding, memory encoding, attention, and information integration across brain regions. Multiple independent research groups have documented disruption of gamma oscillatory activity in Alzheimer's disease, with the degree of disruption correlating with disease severity and cognitive symptom burden. This disruption is observed in both human patients and in transgenic mouse models of Alzheimer's pathology. The mechanism of disruption appears to involve dysfunction of parvalbumin-expressing interneurons, fast-spiking inhibitory neurons that play a critical role in generating gamma rhythms.

The MIT Picower Institute Research Program

The foundational research on 40 Hz sensory entrainment (GENUS: Gamma Entrainment Using Sensory Stimulation) was conducted by Li-Huei Tsai and colleagues at the Picower Institute for Learning and Memory at MIT. Key publications include: Iaccarino et al. (2016), *Nature:* first demonstration that 40 Hz visual flicker reduces amyloid-beta and tau in the visual cortex of 5XFAD mice by approximately 50%, activates microglial phagocytosis, and improves cognitive performance. Martorell et al. (2019), *Cell*: extended the GENUS approach to auditory stimulation, demonstrating that 40 Hz auditory tones produce gamma entrainment in the hippocampus and prefrontal cortex, reduce amyloid-beta and tau in these regions, reduce neuroinflammation, increase synaptic protein levels, and improve spatial memory in mouse models. Combined visual and auditory stimulation produced effects across a broader network than either modality alone.

Human Clinical Research

Cimenser et al. (2021), *Alzheimer's and Dementia: Translational Research and Clinical Interventions*: a human study using combined 40 Hz visual and auditory stimulation in patients with mild Alzheimer's disease over six months. Key findings included significantly reduced brain atrophy in the entorhinal cortex, hippocampus, and other memory-critical regions compared to controls, as well as better preservation of functional connectivity between brain regions and better performance on cognitive assessments. Cognito Therapeutics has conducted Phase 2 clinical trials of combined 40 Hz visual and auditory stimulation in Alzheimer's disease, with interim results showing favorable safety profiles and signals of cognitive benefit in early-stage disease.

PEMF Research Relevant to Cognitive Function

Beyond the 40 Hz entrainment literature, pulsed electromagnetic field therapy has its own substantial research history relevant to neurological and cognitive applications. FDA clearance for PEMF in bone healing was granted in 1979. Subsequent research has examined PEMF's effects on neuroinflammation, neuroprotection, depression, anxiety, and sleep quality. The proposed cellular mechanisms, increased transmembrane voltage and enhanced ATP production, have been demonstrated in multiple in vitro and in vivo studies. ATP production increases of up to 500% following PEMF exposure have been documented in peer-reviewed literature.

A Note on the Current State of the Evidence

The scientific community studying 40 Hz stimulation and PEMF for cognitive applications is active, growing, and producing increasingly rigorous research. The foundational preclinical evidence is strong and well-replicated. Early human evidence is promising and directionally consistent. The definitive large-scale, double-blind, randomized controlled trials that would constitute gold-standard clinical evidence are either ongoing or remain to be conducted. Clinicians and administrators evaluating this evidence should apply the same contextual standards they apply to other emerging evidence-based interventions in geriatric care: assessing the quality of the available evidence, the risk profile of the intervention, and the magnitude of the unmet need.

APPENDIX D

Resources and Next Steps

The following resources are available for facilities and individuals who wish to learn more, evaluate the clinical evidence independently, or apply for the BlueVibe pilot program.

The Facility Pilot Program

The BlueVibe pilot program is a structured 30- to 45-day evaluation designed for memory care facilities. It includes a ten-device system (sufficient to support twenty to forty or more residents daily), pre- and post-assessment resources using the PROMIS Cognitive Function scale, staff orientation materials, and a structured outcome summary report at the conclusion of the pilot. The pilot investment is $1,749. Facilities that proceed to wholesale adoption following the pilot receive pricing that is more than 50% below retail. To apply for a pilot program, visit the BlueVibe page on the Resona Health website.

The Phase 1 Clinical Study

The complete BlueVibe Phase 1 study report, including full methodology, data tables, statistical analysis, and participant feedback, is available on the Resona Health website under the research tab: **Resona.Health** or **ResonaHealth.com.** The study was conducted in 2025-2026 and represents the first completed clinical investigation of BlueVibe's effects on cognitive function in a real-world population.

Resona Health

Resona Health is a technology-driven wellness company focused on developing next-generation, non-invasive therapeutic devices based on principles of frequency, resonance, and bioelectrical signaling. The company's product ecosystem includes VIBE, VaguVibe, BlueVibe, and additional emerging frequency-based therapeutic devices. Information about the full product line, the company's research platform, and its engineering approach is available at resona.health.

Contact and Application

For pilot program applications, wholesale pricing inquiries, clinical study documentation, and facility support:

resona.health/bluevibe-cognitive-support-system

About Mark L. Fox

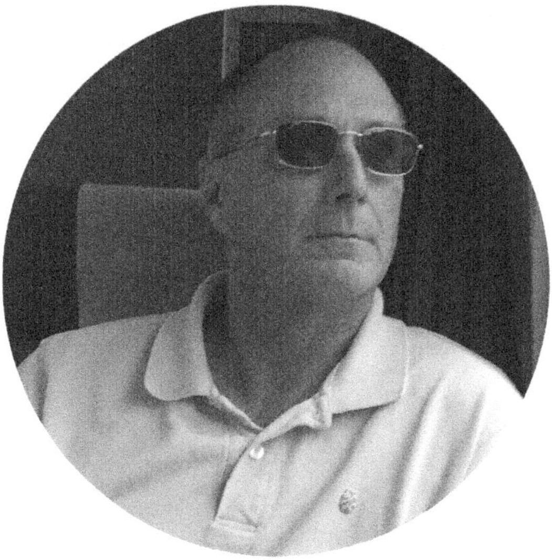

Mark L. Fox is the Founder and CEO of Resona Health and inventor of the BlueVibe cognitive support system. A former NASA Space Shuttle Chief Engineer, Fox left aerospace to apply precision engineering discipline to human wellness. He is an entrepreneur, scientist, author, and speaker whose work spans frequency-based therapy, bioelectromagnetics, and the future of non-invasive care. A hot air balloonist for 35 years who built his own airplane, he lives in Florida.

What Mark's Clients Are Saying About Bluevibe...

"Helping my sleep every night without taking melatonin."

– Flora W.

"It's simple to use. I also believe it has helped me to dream and remember dreams."

– Carolyn H.

"Better concentration. Better sleep. More dreams."

– Christine S.

"It's easy."

– Gary W.

"Edema swelling in feet has reduced considerably."

– Mark S.

"My vivid dreams."

– Mark S.

"Hope for improvement."

– Paula S.

"Convenience and peaceful feeling."

– Amber D.

"It has helped me stay out of the dark places in my mind."

– Amber D.

"I have noticed an improvement in my clarity of thinking and vocabulary words."

– Bonny F.

"I just want to repeat that the clarity and the depth of my thinking have improved. My memory has improved somewhat. However, I do want to say that I had a severe concussion two years ago when I took a fall skiing at 30 miles an hour."

– Bonny F.

"Seemed to brighten my mood."

– Ron J.

"Very convenient and easy."

– Michael H.

"I feel like the short-term memory was lengthened, so instead of forgetting things in about five or ten minutes, it is more like hours and even the next day. Also, my mood improved."

– Michael H.

"Ease of use, improved sleep."

– Jeffry P.

"My wife has advanced dementia. One of her disturbing symptoms is aggressive behavior, like slamming doors and general agitation. Daily use of the BlueVibe seems to have reduced the intensity, frequency, and duration of these behaviors. I would estimate it to be approximately 40%. For myself, as her caregiver, that is a very large blessing. I have more patience and sleep more deeply."

– Jeffry P.

"How easy, inconspicuous, and comfortable it is to use."

– John M.

"I slept very well, and it seems I had better concentration."

– Diane D.

"This was a very positive experience."

– Diane D.

"I think it helped with my sleep and focus."

– Robert M.

"I have been calmer and sleeping better."

– Linda C.

"Easy to use and relaxing."

– Thomas B.

"I noticed better clarity and less stress."

– Susan R.

"Improved sleep and mood."

– Nancy P.

"It gave me more energy during the day."

– James K.

"I felt more focused while using it."

– Barbara T.

"The therapy was simple and effective."

– William F.

"I enjoyed using it and felt more relaxed."

– Karen L.

"I experienced more vivid dreams and deeper sleep."

– Patricia G.

Made in the USA
Monee, IL
13 September 2026

62981878R00059